I0791602

Natural Cancer Cure

How I beat Cancer through Diet and Herbs and found a lifetime of HEALTH and HOPE!

ISBN: 9781976975295

Health, Hope and Herbs

By Russ Lawson
Certified Herbalist - School of Natural
Healing

Dedication:

This book is dedicated to my wife Melody, the love of my life and my partner for the past 51 years on this every changing and challenging journey we call life. Without her encouragement and support I would never have gone on to study Herbal Medicine or write this book. She encouraged me to do both and for this I thank and love her, she is my inspiration!

A REQUST FOR YOU:

Each of us who are Amazon Kindle Authors struggle to make our way in the thousands of book provided here. It would really, really help if you could take a few minutes and leave feedback in the "**Write a Customer Review**" section on my book page. (It's to the right of the box with the stars on the top.

Thanks in advance for your help!
Russ Lawson

Disclaimer:

I have to be up front with you and let you know that ***Federal Regulations prohibits me*** from claiming that herbal products or supplements will cure any disease.

Also, understand that I strongly recommend that you spend time with your health care professional before using any herb, supplement or any other product that claims to be of health benefit.

You can choose to ignore this advice, but you do so at your own risk. My only purpose in ***Health, Hope and Herbs***, is to share what has benefited me and others. Also, understand that each and every one of us is different, our bodies don't react the same all of the time, what works for me, may not work as well for you or you may have a undesired reaction and some of the herbs available are quite strong and some can have a toxic effect on your body. So, proceed with whatever you choose to do with caution. Do your research, check with professionals because after all you literally do hold your life in your own hands.

Let me say that I completely understand that the use of Herbs and Supplements are not for everyone. I have encountered many skeptics in this area of alternative medicine and that's alright. Everyone is entitled to their own opinion and what they choose to believe, however if you are reading this, you must have some question as to whether their might actually be a glimmer of hope for better health. That's why I chose to write, *Health, Hope and Herbs*.

PLEASE NOTE: Although I do hold a couple of PhD's and am a Certified Herbalist, **I am not a medical doctor**, so please bear that in mind as you read this book. (*Please note this is for informational purposes only and not intended as medical advice. Check with your own doctor before trying any health remedy.*)

Russ Lawson

Chapter One

My Journey to better health and hope through herbs

I consider life a journey and sometimes I view it as part of my <u>unexpected adventure</u> on this road called life. You never know 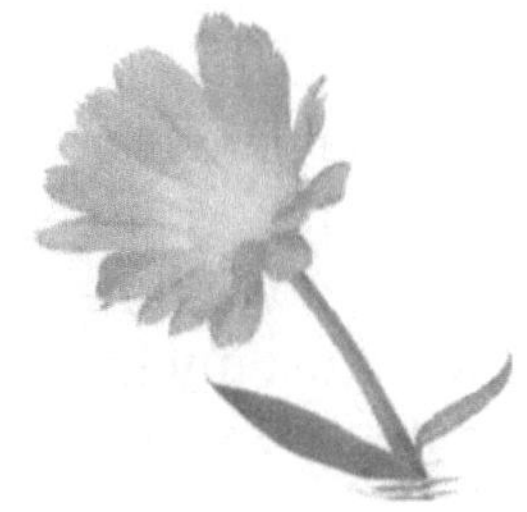 which way the road is going to twist and turn and you are always presented with choices as the road branches. I pray that your journey can be filled with hope no matter what problems or health issues challenge you.

As I begin, let me tell you a little about myself and my health. I am 70 years old and take no prescription medicine and work a full time 40 hour a week in a physically demanding job. Also I have had no major health issues to date, which I like to attribute to my use of herbs and supplements.

Now having said that I also don't take any prescriptions, but let me explain why just a little further. The bottom line as they say; is that I don't need any. One of the biggest problems for folks as they age is their blood pressure. My blood pressure normally is 125/72 with an average pulse of 60. Another issue is diabetes, for me my numbers are great as well as my cholesterol levels.

I also don't have arthritics which is almost amazing for "mature" people in our society. Occasionally I'll have an ache or pain and I try to adjust my herbs or minerals to deal with that.

Could that be just a "genetics thing"? I don't know I am not a geneticist. I do know that before my father's death he was crippled with two types of arthritics. He had both knees replaced, his toes straightened and his hands were so deformed he could hardly use them.

My 91 year old mother also struggles with arthritis, and both of them were or are on several prescription drugs for various issues. So genetics… I'm not learned in that area, but in this book, I deal with Health, Hope and Herbs and I'll share some of my thoughts on the subject.

As I share my journey to better understand herbs as an alternative medicine, understand it was not a short journey. In fact, it began almost 30 years ago and is still continuing.

The Beginning

In 1993 we were living in Kenya, East Africa working and traveling several times per week in the rural (bush) villages. The roads were always in terrible condition (when there were roads). One particular day we were traveling to a village and the driver hit a terrible pot hole. It was so bad that even wearing a seat belt my head bounced off of the roof of the vehicle.

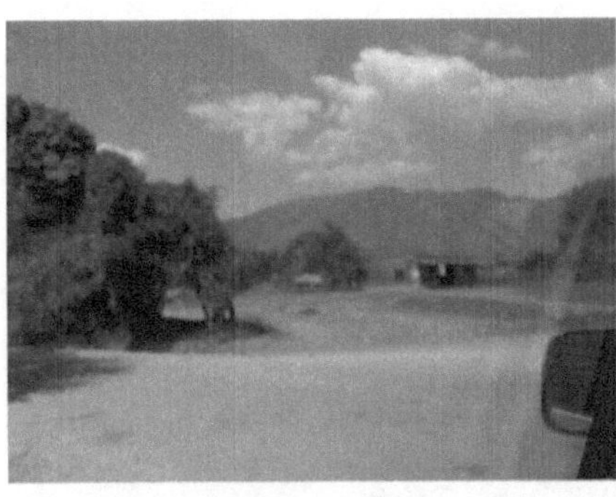

The next day I could hardly move for the pain in my lower neck and arm. We had a good friend who happened to be our family doctor also. He was an Orthopedic Surgeon who had a family practice; he was originally from India and had trained in Great Britain.

He gave me the pain medicine and muscle relaxers and put my arm in a sling to immobilize it. He also ordered X-rays which showed I had a collapsed disk in my lower neck. The basic treatment was to take it easy and give my body a chance to heal itself.

After several weeks and no improvement, (still in pain, arm still in the sling), my doctor friend asked if I would be open to trying something different, an "alternative medicine" treatment. By that time I was willing to try just about anything, so was ready to hear him out.

The doctor said he had begun studying homeopathic medicine and thought he found a treatment which might help. So, I agreed to try this new method of healing, with which I really was unfamiliar. He said he would have to order the medicine from India and my new journey began.

Homeopathic Medicine

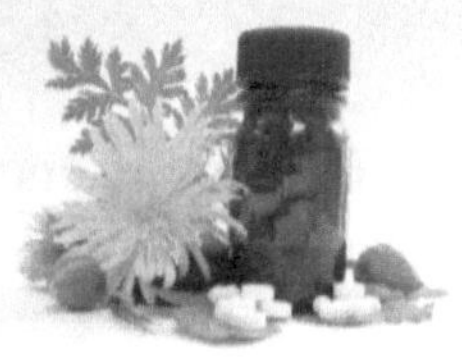

"Homeopathy, or homeopathic medicine, is a medical philosophy and practice based on the idea that the body has the ability to heal itself. Homeopathy was founded in the late 1700s in Germany and has been widely practiced throughout Europe. Homeopathic medicine views symptoms of illness as normal responses of the body as it attempts to regain health.

Homeopathy is based on the idea that "like cures like." That is, if a substance causes a symptom in a healthy person, giving the person a very small amount of the same substance may cure the illness. In theory, a homeopathic dose enhances the body's normal healing and self-regulatory processes." (Definition from WebMD.com)

The medicine arrived and we began treatment which consisted of taking a tiny sugar pill saturated in the homeopathically distilled medicine, placing it under my tongue and letting it dissolve a couple of times a day.

The results were surprising, even amazing you could say. I started to have relief for the pain in a few days and within two weeks I was no longer wearing the sling and in another week or so I was back to my normal routine.

What was the homeopathic medicine? I have no idea and my doctor/ friend died a few years ago so I can't ask him. There are homeopathic practitioners throughout almost every country. You can do a search of the Internet to find one near you, but you can check here also, http://homeopathyusa.org.

This book is directed at giving you hope and "I hope" I am successful. I can't promise that anyone else will have the same success with this type of treatment as did I, but my greatest desire is that you will find something on your journey which will help you have a better life.

This was the beginning… my introduction into a world which contained medical treatment outside of my previous experiences. I began a journey towards understanding a little better that sometimes Alternative Medicine works.

I have several good friends who are medical doctors in my life yet today. I cherish their friendship and their advice, but I also know that they are somewhat skeptical about Alternative Medicine. I understand this completely.

There are a lot of "Quacks" out there trying to sell some "miracle cure," or some "magic potion," which really has only one purpose which is to make money for the seller. Understand this please, I AM NOT SELLING ANYTHING, I am sharing my experiences, the experiences of friends and my many years of knowledge through intense study.

Also, please understand, there are many very honest, very upright, very educated practitioners of Alternative Medicine. Whatever you chose, whoever you choose to go to for advice, check them out thoroughly. Just because someone says they know what they are doing doesn't make it so.

Chapter Two

The Next Branch in My Road - CANCER

We returned from Kenya to the United States and restarted our lives enjoying work, family and especially a new grandson. Things went well for us for a time, but then in 2002 I developed a persistent cough. I went to my doctor who was and still is a close friend. He a thought it was a bronchial infection, (I had been prone to those since returning from Africa), but the cough persisted. He sent me for x-rays and it showed a spot on my right lung.

My doctor was concerned of course and referred me to a lung specialist. The specialist started a whole battery of test, more x-rays, CAT scan, Sonogram and the most conclusive a PET scan. Now just in case you don't know what that is, here is the medical definition:

"Positron emission tomography, also called PET imaging or a PET scan, is a type of nuclear medicine imaging.

Nuclear medicine is a branch of medical imaging that uses small amounts of radioactive material to diagnose and determine the severity of or treat a variety of diseases, including many types of cancers, heart disease, gastrointestinal, endocrine, neurological disorders and other abnormalities within the body. Because nuclear medicine procedures are able to pinpoint molecular activity within the body, they offer the potential to identify disease in its earliest stages as well as a patient's immediate response to therapeutic interventions." (www.radiologyinfo.org).

Basically they put radioactive material in sugar water (glucose) and put it into your blood stream. Cancer cells love sugar, so they gobble it up and then they glow brightly when they take images of your body.

The Results

I remember very clearly the day we did the follow-up visit with the lung specialist. We of course were sent to a consulting room and eventually the doctor came in and said, "***Mr. Lawson, the test show conclusively that you have a cancerous mass in your right lung***". He paused waiting for a response from me; I just looked at him and said, *"OK, what do we do next?"*

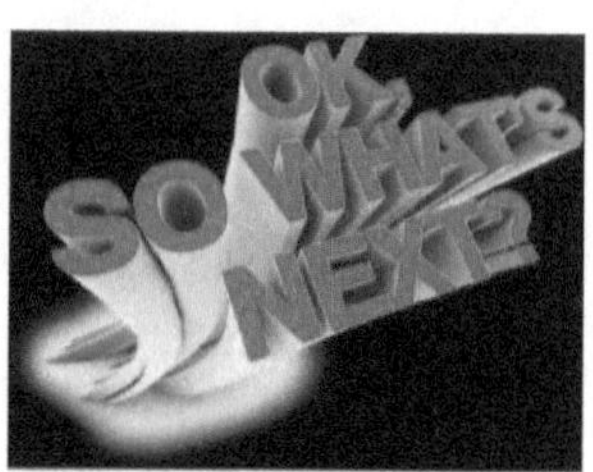

He had kind of a shocked look on his face as he didn't know what to say next. He then said, *"As long as I have been dealing with people no one has ever responded that way."* I suppose he was used to someone breaking down in tears or such, which I can very easily understand. I responded to him, *"Well, God was in control when I came into this room and He still is!"* He didn't quite know what to make of that, but we continued with the consultation. You may get a glimmer of how important my faith is to me.

The results of the tests showed that I had a small mass in my right lung behind my heart. This of course made it a little harder to get to or treat. He of course discussed several methods of treatment and we said we needed to talk and pray about it. (I haven't mentioned it, but I had been a Minister for around 31 years at this time.)

We went home and talked and prayed about it. I told my wife (having been a minster for so long), I had seen so many people exactly where we were at. I had seen them go through the chemo and radiation treatments and the results were a life of misery. Yes, the treatments sometimes were successful, but struggles people had just dealing with all of the side effects didn't interest me. Also the success rates for the treatments at the time were dismal to say the least.

In the end I decided that I would not undergo any of the traditional treatment methods, but I would look into alternative treatment. So, I began yet again a new branch in the road for _my unexpected adventure_, (my first book).

Chapter 3

The Eyologist

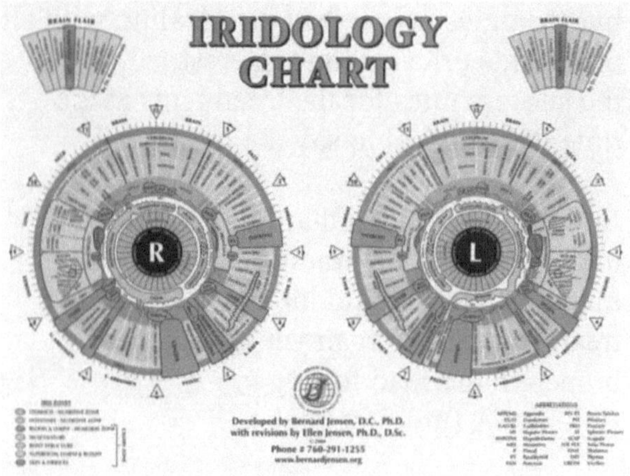

Where to begin? How to begin? Of course I immediately began searching out articles about alternative medicine in relation to cancer. My studies began in earnest when it was something that affected me in such a personal way.

We knew that some friends and fellow church members were involved some way with alternative medicine and herbs, but weren't sure in what way. We approached them and found that they took several herbal compounds themselves, but didn't have a deep understanding of the practice of herbal medicine. During our discussions we did discover that they knew of someone who might be able to help guide me… they knew an Eyologist.

Probably like many of you, we had no idea what an Eyologist was. Here are the basics:

> "An Eyologist is someone who is trained in both the sciences of Iridology and Sclerology. Whereas Iridology involves the assessment of the iris, **Sclerology** or the new term, **Sclera Analysis**, involves the assessment of the lines and various markings in the whites (or sclera) of the eye. Together, the clinical data which can be obtained provides a very accurate and thorough analysis of various organs and systems in the body which are stressed or congested."
> (http://waytogonutrition.com/eyology.htm)

OK, basically the Eyologist is trained to look in your eye and diagnose a problem in your body. Yes, right, I was, as many of you are, totally skeptical, however trying to keep an open mind I made an appointment for a reading. **NOTE:** Because I was a skeptic I did not indicate in anyway why I was there, only that I wanted a reading (a check up). She examined me and when she was done told me she saw a dark mass in my right lung.

WHAT? How could she know that, it took teams of specialist, millions of dollars of specialized equipment and thousands of dollars worth of testing for my doctor tell me the same thing. That's something that kind of shakes your foundation of "What you think you know and understand".

I asked her what she suggested as far as treatment and basically it was things that would cleanse my system. So, this prompted even more in-depth research.

In the mean time I let the lung specialist know that for the present I would not be taking any treatment, only monitoring the situation with regular visits.

As I scoured the Internet I was amazed at how much information there was available on concept of alternative treatment for cancer. Of course much of the information is confusing and undocumented, but if you study enough you learn to cull out the real from the unreal for the most part. After a couple of weeks of study I decided on incorporating a couple of the alternative treatments into my life and began doing that, (I'll share what I did later).

THE RESULTS

Several weeks later and after a few visits to the specialist he convinced me to allow him to remove the mass (tumor) via surgery. I told him I would approve that, but would not take chemotherapy or radiation. So we set the date and began the final tests before surgery. The day before the surgery was scheduled he sent me for a final CAT scan to be followed with a consultation.

I don't think I will ever forget the events of that day. I had the test and went to the specialist office (in the same building). We waited an extra long time for the doctor to come into the consultation room. When he finally came in you could tell from his voice and his demeanor that he was agitated, perhaps frustrated. The first words out of his mouth in a loud and obviously stressed voice were, "***Mr. Lawson, you had cancer and now it's gone and I don't know what happened!***" I replied, "***Would you like for me to tell you.***" His response floored me when he said, "***I don't want to hear it!***" I still haven't understood that comment after all of these years… If there were a way to help patients, without chemo, radiation or surgery, wouldn't you logically, as a doctor, want to know about it?

I have no doubt that he is a good man and a competent doctor, but he was also unwilling to consider anything that was not an accepted, modern medical procedure. In reality, the majority of doctors are not trained in the effectiveness of Alternative Medicine or the use of Herbs to combat illness.

> ***When we talk about Herbal Medicine we are talking about: "the art or practice of using herbs and herbal preparations to maintain health and to prevent, alleviate, or cure disease." (Webster's Dictionary)***

What is considered an Herb by Herbal Practitioners'? An Herb is almost anything that grows. The leaves, seeds, roots and sometimes the stems are used. Some definitions do not include woody plants or stems, but in reality we often use all parts of the plant, including things like the hull of a black walnut. Herbal Practitioners believe that God gave us and intended us to use all of his creation and we continue to search out that which will aid in healing the body from natural means.

Chapter 4

The Road Branches Yet Again…

After my "miracle cure," I continued to read everything I could on herbal and/or alternative medicine. It amazed me (and still does), how the body can many times heal itself when cleansed and given the proper nutrition.

I spent so much time reading and studying that my wife finally told me, (basically), **"Why don't you start studying that stuff at a credible school."** So, I began searching for just that, there are several really good schools for natural medicine, but I ended up registering with the country's highest rated Herbal school and one of the oldest, The School of Natural Healing, founded by Dr. John Christopher in 1953. Dr. Christopher was a Medical Doctor and also practiced Herbal Medicine. Dr. Christopher became a Master Herbalist in 1946 after completing course work under Dr. H. Knowles at Dominion Herbal College in Vancouver, British Columbia. In 1948 he received his Naturopathic Doctor degree from the Institute of Drugless Therapy in Tama, Iowa. I will be sharing links to several of his book later.

So, I undertook a new endeavor, traveling on a new branch in the road so to speak. I obtained my basic certification as a Family Herbalist (a Junior college degree if you will), and am still in the midst of studies to become a Master Herbalist at this time.

If you take a look at the school's website you will see that the number of courses required seem almost overwhelming, but if you choose this road, it is one you will never regret.

Chapter 5

Let's begin with the big "C", Cancer.

The American Cancer Society predicts: "*in 2017, there will be an estimated* **1,688,780** *new cancer cases diagnosed and* **600,920** *cancer deaths in the US*".

What I would do if I found that I had cancer…. Again….. (Any cancer)? If you are like most of us who have faced that question you will begin to seek out answers. You will put all of your time, all of your effort and much of your money into trying to beat this terrible disease. That's what I did and I want to share some of my findings.

To begin with let me say that there is no "one treatment" for cancer. There are many things that work to tame this deadly disease, which is in direct contrast to the prevailing mentality regarding the matter. I have been researching cancer treatments and cures for about 20 years and I know as you approach the search for alternative treatments you will be overwhelmed. We all want some guarantee, some miracle cure that is guaranteed to succeed. I will warn you up front that there are plenty of people in this world who will be glad to claim "A Cure," and take your money as quickly as they can get it from you.

I have an antique bottle with the label still attached and some liquid inside. The label claims it is "DR. Johnson's Snake Oil," (yes really), and it claims to cure a great number of ailments. I am not selling "Snake Oil," in fact I'm not selling anything at all. I will recommend many things in this book, but I urge you to be fastidious in doing your own research as to how any herb or supplement might help or effect you personally.

What I am trying to do here is to share just a few things and encourage you to continue to research the available treatments on your own. Each person's body is unique, their circumstances are unique, their physical environment is unique; therefore each person will most likely respond differently to any give approach to dealing with the problem of cancer. (Note: in the material below, I have placed many of the hyperlinks in the text which will allow you to just click on them (or type them in the paperback edition), and continue your research, perhaps giving you more information to share with your doctor).

<u>What I did</u>

First of all, I didn't make a lot of changes in my diet and we already had a pretty clean diet, however through the years I have made more changes. If you are not eating a diet of lots of organic vegetables and certified clean (hormone and antibiotic free meats), you need to begin doing so. There is a great book out titled: **"Eat to live"** by Dr. Joel Fuhrman which I highly recommend. It just may convince you to watch what you eat more closely. He is convinced as am I, that almost all disease is a result of what we put into or on our bodies.

Second, I stopped using any artificial sweeteners. It has been proven many times over that these do tremendous damage to your body and many actually encourage cancer in the body.

Third, I cut back on the amount of sugar I used or products containing sugar, (cancer thrives on sugar), and many food products contain "high fructose corn syrup" which is especially bad for you, no matter what the commercials on television say.

Fourth, I became very conscious of reading labels and avoiding products with additives in them, especially processed foods of any kind. **Note**: This is especially true of soda pop, diet or regular, they are terribly bad for you. I also would recommend switching to distilled water rather than tap water. We eventually purchased a water distiller and now distill all of our drinking water.

Fifth, my studies taught me that your skin is the largest single organ in your body. I became very conscious regarding what products I put on my skin, especially soap, deodorants, toothpastes, shampoo, hand sanitizer, etc. Your skin will absorb all of the dangerous chemicals you place on it, so be careful.

If you are using after shave, soaps, body lotions, and deodorants that contain fragrances, then you are exposing yourself to chemicals that can cause many problems for your body. More than 3,000 chemicals are used in so-called fragrances, and two-thirds of them have not been safety tested. In addition, some of them have been linked to allergic reactions and hormone disruption.

I know it is not what you expect because of what is on the label's, but even "fragranced free " products often contain potentially toxic substances such as parabens, petroleum, and phthalates and are definitely bad for your body.

I make my own hand soap, hand sanitizer, etc., but you can find good clean products at your local health supply/food store. I purchase an all natural bar soap from our local health food store, simply because it is much easier than making my own bar soap at this time. You will find that in almost every case the folks who work at the health food stores are knowledgeable and extremely helpful in talking to you about the products available in their stores. Generally they are a good reference source.

What Herbs and Supplements did I take to combat my cancer?

I want to encourage you to visit your local health food store to purchase any of the products mentioned here. However if you can't find them I am providing other sources with which you can check.

Liquid Minerals from American Youngevity. They have changed the name to "Ultra Body Toddy", but it can be ordered from <u>American Youngevity</u> or phone **(800) 982-3189**.

Why this product? After my research I learned that most of us don't get the proper vitamins and minerals in our systems through our food. Yes, I know that you take vitamin/mineral and supplements, but most of the time they are in the form of hard compacted tablets which don't dissolve in your system and pass straight through your digestive system. The liquid minerals insure that you get what you need into your system to build your system and help fight cancer or any other disease. Vitamin D is especially necessary for healing cancer and in particular Lung Cancer.

Stabilized Rice Bran

Now this product is widely available through the Internet or Health Food Stores, it wasn't when I began. It is nutrient rich and contains over 100 anti-oxidants. You need to build your immune system and this is an excellent way to do this.

The benefits of this product was initially discovered in India. Rice Bran, (the outer hull), is milled off of the rice to present an attractive product. Researchers discovered that mothers in India would go to the mill and gather the discarded Rice Bran and make a broth from it and give it to their sick children. The children, more often than not would recover. When they began to research the reason, they found that Rice Bran was filled with good things. As is often done, we discard the most beneficial part of the plant because we don't like the look, the texture or the taste.

Boost Immunity

"Abnormal cells, bacteria, and viruses proliferate in our bodies all the time, but normally the immune system annihilates them before they have a chance to develop into illness, disease or cancer.

The immune system is a complex network coordinating the activities that protect us from harmful microbial invaders (bacteria, viruses, fungi and parasites) and stop abnormal cell proliferation. This system protects us from all types of illness and disease. But it can be weakened by nutritional deficiencies, prolonged illness and inflammation, and by the carcinogens, dangerous metals, poisons, toxins and stress we are exposed to every day.

When a person has a weakened immune system, even a simple cold or flu can escalate and become a life-threatening illness. Having a strong immune system is the best defense against illness and disease. Nutritionally strengthening and supporting the immune system is essential, especially after the age of 50 because the body's natural defenses decline with age.

Sterols and Sterolins (found in plants) are great immune supporters. They help the immune system stop cancer, kill bacteria, destroy viruses and slow down the aging process. They have also been shown to keep patients infected with the HIV virus from developing AIDS. Stabilized rice bran has high concentrations of Sterolins and Phytosterols that have demonstrated potent antiviral and antibacterial effects.

Stabilized rice bran also contains the following immune system helpers:

1. Polysaccharides (known to improve immune function)
2. Gamma Oryzanol and other phytonutrients that increase

immune response and reduce pro-inflammatory cytokines

3. Omegas 3, 6 & 9 fatty acids and Tocopherols & Tocotrienols that have been shown to suppress auto anti-DNA antibodies
4. CoQ10 which is a known immune booster routinely recommended as part of the treatment for people suffering from: Cardiovascular Disease, Parkinson's Disease, Muscular Dystrophy, Cancer, Diabetes Mellitus, Infertility, AIDS, Asthma, Thyroid Disorders, and Periodontal Disease
5. Alpha Lipoic Acid which is extremely effective against oxidative stress and free radical destruction.

Lower Cancer Risk

Cancer is now the leading cause of death globally. It is estimated that cancer will kill 84 million people in the next ten years. While the causes of cancer are complex, it is well known that certain things can lower the risk of getting it.

The most important recommendations are to avoid toxins and eat healthy foods. Stabilized rice bran has many nutrients that are known to help protect against cancer". (WebND)

What I would add

As I said above, I am continually studying and learning. I am currently enrolled in The School of Natural Healing in Utah where I plan on eventually having a certification as a Master Herbalist.

Recently I read the report below that I want to share here. If I were diagnosed with cancer again, I would follow this regime also.

NOTE 1: If you decide to try some of these herbal products they will not interfere with any current medication you are taking, but will assist in your recovery from the condition.

NOTE 2: I am not a doctor and cannot prescribe or recommend treatment; I can only share what I have used and done myself. (*Please note this is for informational purposes only and not* *intended as medical advice. Check with your own doctor before trying out any health remedies.*)

First, I would cleanse my system.

Far too often our intestinal track has a build up of old fecal matter. It actually lines the nooks and crannies of our intestines much like spreading a coating of plaster on them. If left there it will harden. It is impossible for your body to get the nutrients it needs if your intestines can't do the job God designed them to do.

You can go about this more than one way of course, but the School of Natural Healing recommends a 3 day course of cleansing if you can physically do it. This is three days of drinking an 8oz glass of all natural prune juice in the morning followed by as much all natural apple juice (not the stuff at the grocery which is mostly sugar and water) and distilled water as you can drink comfortably. Anytime you feel hungry drink another glass of juice or distilled water. You can also begin and speed up the process by taking Dr. Christopher's Lower Bowel Formula, which is an all natural, and gentle, laxative. This formula is available at: http://www.drchristophersherbshop.com or by calling (888) 327-4372.

Next I would add as much fresh juice to my diet as I could

Juicing is one of the best ways to get the maximum amount of nutrients and antioxidants into your system. Though you need to be carful of the types of juice you make or purchase. Juices can raise your blood sugar. As a great reference though check out http://www.chrisbeatcancer.com.

Apple Juice, Most are familiar with the old 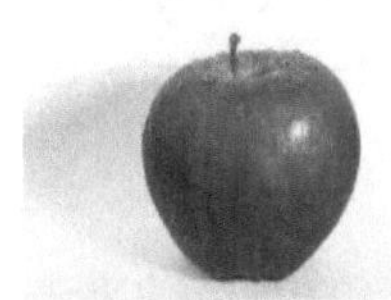 saying, "An apple a day keeps the Doctor away," and there really is some truth to that idea. One of the best blood purifiers known is the apple. Dr. Edward Shook states, "*There is no other agent or herb that can compare with the apple tree... Its abundance of Nascent oxygen compound is probably the main reason why it is such a precious food, blood purifier and unfailing remedy for so many forms of diseases*." For this reason, I would drink lots of apple juice. If you can get fresh un-pasteurized apple cider it will work well also.

Carrot Juice is also excellent for many of the same reasons and some use only 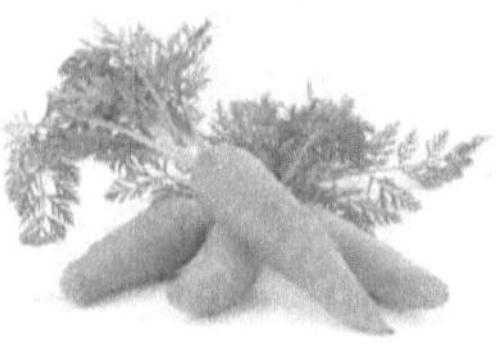 carrot juice very effectively, however drinking this much carrot juice may actually cause your skin to take on an orange hue if continued long enough. And personally I (and others I talked with), get tired of the taste really quickly.

You may want to vary what you drink. Drink Carrot juice for the first day, then apple juice for the next, perhaps grape the third. You need to do what will allow you to continue feeding your body what it needs to treatment itself.

How much: You will want to drink at least a quart per day.

NOTE: Do not purchase pre-bottled juice in the grocery; it is rare to find a truly "Natural" juice in a grocery store. I recommend that you purchase a juicing machine of some type and make your own juice. You might be able to purchase all natural juice from your health food store, but almost all of these have been pasteurized (heated) which destroys most of the effectiveness of the juice.

Chew your juice

OK, Yes I know how silly that sounds, but it is necessary and here is why. The saliva that your mouth produces is one of the main ingredients necessary for your digestive system to work properly. Your mouth has been called "the mixing bowl" for your body. When you chew your food your saliva is mixed into the food and it begins processing the food so that your body can harvest the nutrients contained in the food.

How do you chew your juice? Simply hold it in you mouth for a few seconds and swish it around. This will allow the saliva to mix with the juice and allow you to get the maximum benefits from the juice you drink.

Chapter 6

Cancer - High-dose vitamin C injections shown to annihilate cancer

For those with advanced cancer I would really consider this as a place to begin as well as adding some of the other things suggested. The problem with this approach is finding a doctor or clinic which will agree to administer it. From what I have read, you will have to be persistent and force the issue for the doctor to agree as most think of it as quackery. You need to let them know that it is your body and this is what you want and that it will do no harm even if it does not work. I had one friend who had advanced cancer and tried to get this procedure, but by the time they found someone to administer the treatment she was too weak to take it and died shortly after.

(The following by Ethan A. Huff, staff writer NaturalNews.com)

(From NaturalNews.com) Groundbreaking new research on the cancer-fighting potential of vitamin C has made the pages of the peer-reviewed journal *Science Translational Medicine*. A team of researchers from the University of Kansas reportedly tested the effects of vitamin C

given in high doses intravenously on a group of human subjects and found that it effectively eradicates cancer cells while leaving healthy cells intact.

"Patients are looking for safe and low-cost choices in their management of cancer," stated Dr. Jeanne Drisko, a co-author of the study, to *BBC News* concerning the findings. "Intravenous vitamin C has that potential based on our basic science research and early clinical data."

Researchers admit more human trials on intravenous vitamin C unlikely because drug companies cannot patent vitamins

"Because vitamin C has no patent potential, its development will not be supported by pharmaceutical companies," says Qi Chen, lead author of the new study. "We believe that the time has arrived for research agencies to vigorously support thoughtful and meticulous clinical trials with intravenous vitamin C."

"[A]scorbate is processed by the body in different ways when administered orally versus intravenously," writes Heidi Ledford for *Nature* about this commonly misunderstood variance. The medical-industrial complex, it turns out, intentionally corrupts the conversation on vitamin C by convoluting the distinct effects of these very different delivery routes.

"Oral doses [of vitamin C] act as antioxidants, protecting cells from damage caused by reactive compounds that contain oxygen. But vitamin C given intravenously can have the opposite effect by promoting the formation of one of those compounds: hydrogen peroxide. Cancer cells are particularly susceptible to damage by such reactive oxygen-containing compounds."

Sources for this article include:
http://www.nature.com
http://www.bbc.co.uk
http://lpi.oregonstate.edu
http://science.naturalnews.com

Here is another prospective regarding using Vitamin C Therapy

IV Vitamin C therapy: A cancer perspective

by Jonathan Landsman (NaturalNews.com)

"Cancer patients need to understand the danger of vitamin C deficiencies - especially when looking to overcome a cancer diagnosis. In truth, most people suffering with any chronic degenerative disease are vitamin C deficient. Sadly, it's a fact that Western medicine refuses to recognize due to the influence of the pharmaceutical industry.

Cancer patients find relief with IV vitamin C therapy:

Over 40 years ago, Nobel laureate Linus Pauling and Ewan Cameron, MD, a Scottish cancer surgeon, demonstrated the effectiveness of 10,000 mg of vitamin C, per day, to reverse cancer in thirteen patients - that were left to die by conventional medicine

Western medicine continues to ignore the truth about vitamin C and natural cancer therapies

Excited about the healing power of vitamin C, Linus Pauling went to the National Cancer Institute, where he was systematically ignored and ridiculed. To this day, if you visit any conventional cancer website (controlled by the pharmaceutical industry) you'll discover a complete lack of honesty about the effectiveness of vitamin C for cancer patients.

If you're an open-minded healthcare professional, I suggest you investigate the magnificent work of biochemist Irwin Stone, *The Healing Factor*; Linus Pauling and Ewan Cameron, M.D., *Cancer and Vitamin C*; plus many other great vitamin C experts like, Drs. William McCormick, Fredrick Klenner, Thomas E. Levy and Ronald Hunninghake. (And, yes, there are many more medical professionals)

Visit: http://www.naturalhealth365.com for more information"

"Three vitamin C - unfounded beliefs that hurt or kill cancer patients - every day (NaturalNews.com)

Untruth #1: 'There is no evidence that vitamin C works'. Are you kidding me? A recent search, in PubMed, reveals well over 50,000 studies on vitamin C and literally dozens of remarkable studies revealing the power of vitamin C to treatment diseases, such as, 60 out of 60 cases of polio; 327 out of 327 cases of shingles - in 3 days; 7 out of 7 cases of rheumatic fever and, of course, to help cancer patients to thrive under 'incurable' situations. Ignoring this truth ought to be classified as a criminal behavior by Western medicine.

Untruth #2: 'Vitamin C is not safe.' Let's be

perfectly clear, vitamin C has been successfully used - since the 1940's - without a single confirmed report of any dose doing any significant harm to any individual. Yet, according to the Journal of the American Medical Association, 106,000 patients died in hospitals, in 1994, from 'legally-prescribed', carefully-supervised medications and that number hasn't changed for 30 years. That's over 3 million deaths from approved drugs and they have the nerve to say vitamin C isn't safe? Now that borders on insanity. (Wouldn't you agree?)

Untruth #3: 'If vitamin C worked, we'd all be using it.' For a physician to be so convinced (and say) that vitamin C doesn't work - without ever administering a single vitamin C infusion is truly negligent. According to **Thomas E. Levy, M.D., JD**, "I've personally witnessed hundreds of "medical miracles" as a response to high-dose vitamin C."

The conventionally-trained medical community does not want you to learn the truth about vitamin C.

Do some research on **Ronald Hunninghake, M.D**., an internationally recognized expert in IV vitamin C. Discover the healing power of IV vitamin C for cancer plus many other diseases

Dr. Hunninghake is the Chief Medical Officer of the Olive W. Garvey Center for Healing Arts, the clinical division of the Riordan Clinic. A 1976 graduate of the University Of Kansas School Of Medicine, Dr. Hunninghake has devoted his career to the emerging paradigm of Self Care: the patient as an informed medical partner.

From the first days of medical school, he has sought to find new ways of encouraging his patients to take better care of themselves, form new and sustainable habits of health, and to assume greater responsibility in their own health care. He was named the 2011 Orthomolecular Doctor of the Year by the International Society for Orthomolecular Medicine and is a 2013 inductee into the Orthomolecular Hall of Fame.

The truth about vitamin C gets revealed! Despite the lies and scientific fraud, people are waking up to the power of high dose vitamin C to promote healing. One of the most powerful antioxidants on the planet, vitamin C helps to destroy cancer cells and boost immune function - at the same time. Research: The 'Riordan IVC protocol' for cancer patients." (Natural.News.com)
A couple of websites at which you might want to look:
http://www.naturalhealth365.com
http://www.chrisbeatcancer.com

Chapter 7

Another one of the many treatments

What if I told you carrots treatment cancer?
By Paul Fassa

"Ann Cameron, an author of 15 children's books, treated her Stage 4 cancer with carrot juice only. She states, "I believe from personal experience that carrots can treatment cancer - and rapidly, without chemotherapy, radiation, or other dietary changes."

On June 6, 2012, Ann had surgery for Stage 3 colon cancer. She had decided against chemotherapy and actually started feeling better, until about November 6, 2012.

A routine follow-up CT scan indicated lung cancer. She was diagnosed with Stage 4 colon cancer which had metastasized to the lungs. Her doctor predicted a two to three year life expectancy.

She was advised that radiation would be

useless, and chemotherapy was recommended, but it wouldn't extend her life.

Five Pounds of Carrots Juiced Daily

Ann embarked on an intensive research campaign to find an alternative protocol that would heal her.

In her search, she came across a man who had treated his cancer with nothing but carrots. His name was Ralph Cole, and he had treated his small squamous cell cancer (on his neck) by drinking 5 pounds of carrots juiced daily. Ralph shared his carrot curing protocol freely with anyone who would listen.

On November 17, Ann began a daily regimen of 5 pounds of juiced carrots (one quart to a quart and one-third daily). Ann juiced in the morning, drank a glass and then refrigerated the rest, which she finished off throughout the day. Ann faithfully continued juicing five pounds of carrots daily.

The only exception was every month or so when she was traveling she would forgo the carrot juice for three or four days consecutively.

Ann had no chemo, no radiation and no other dietary modifications except carrot juice. She continued eating meat and sometimes indulged in various unhealthy foods, including ice cream.

A PET scan (Positron Emission Tomography) on November 27, 2012, corroborated the earlier CT scan: "Enlarged swollen lymph nodes, containing two 1 inch long by 1/4 inch diameter rapidly growing tumors between the lungs."

On January 7, 2013, after eight weeks of daily carrot juicing, another follow-up CT scan revealed that the cancerous tumors had stopped growing, there had been some tumor shrinkage and there was a reduction in swollen lymph nodes.

CT Scans

March 2013: The cancer had not grown. No new cancer, no swollen lymph nodes, and tumors continued shrinking. July 30, 2013: The cancer was gone! All swollen cancerous lymph nodes had returned to normal.

Summary

• Two weeks of daily carrot juicing: no improvement.
• Eight weeks of juicing: the cancer stopped growing and tumors began shrinking.
• Four months of juicing: all the lymph

nodes in the lungs were normal.
• Eight months of juicing: all the cancer was gone!

Carrots and Cancer Research

Falcarinol is an antioxidant found in carrots and has proven anticancer properties. Researchers in the UK and Denmark reduced cancerous tumors by 1/3 in mice and rats with lab induced cancers.

Additionally, a human study found that consumption of carrot juice increased blood levels of carotenoids in breast cancer survivors. The researchers believe that increased carotenoid blood levels acts as a cancer preventive." (Natural News)

Sources for more information include:
http://www.chrisbeatcancer.com
http://www.chrisbeatcancer.com
http://cancerisover.blogspot.com
http://www.alive.com
http://treatmentcancercells.com
http://www.carrotmuseum.co.uk

About the author: Paul Fassa: You can visit his blog at
http://healthmaven.blogspot.com

** NOTE FROM RUSS LAWSON ABOUT CARROT JUICE TREATMENT:

I have tried juicing and drinking carrot juice. While it can be done, it is difficult, you get tired of carrots rather quickly, but if you are motivated by you cancer, you can do it. But remember, this is only one of the many natural treatments out there. A change in diet is the main thing that will make a difference, adding the right herbs, fruits and vegetables will change your life.

Understand that these are NOT "overnight" treatments, they take time to work, but will restore your body if given time. Also understand they are not for everyone and they are not guaranteed to rid your body of cancer. Sometimes a person's body is just too filled with a disease to effectively fight it off or sometimes the body is just simply too weak to respond to whatever treatment you may decide to partake in to deal with your problem.

Chapter 8

STREGNTHEN YOUR IMMUNE SYSTEM

In reality the key to having better health is to strengthen your immune system. If you have a strong immune system, your body will be able to naturally fight off pretty much any disease from allergies to colds to cancer.

I'll make a few suggestions that should be of benefit to most of us.

Once again, let me stress that you must clean up your diet. One of the most damaging things about our present society is that "Quick and Easy" foods are the way most people survive. The general rule for good health is if it comes in a box don't eat it. I know that the idea of "cooking from scratch" (starting with basic ingredients and making it yourself), is almost a thing of the past, but if you want to live long and healthy lives it is a must.

Have you wondered about the increase of illness, disease and obesity? The main cause is the fact that something like 75% of all meals eaten in the United States come from boxes or a fast food restaurant. If you want to be healthy you can't do that on a regular basis. Each of us need to eat a healthy diet filled with lots of raw, fresh, organic produce, full of enzymes and vitamins. You will want to avoid any product that says it contains GMO's, Corn Syrup or sugar.

You may or may not have heard this, but you need to stop eating processed meats, lunch meats, hotdogs, etc. They have so many preservatives and chemicals in them especially Nitrates that destroy your immune system and cause disease. Companies are now producing lunch meats, bacon and ham without any nitrates. Most are labeled as "Uncured, Organic or Hormone Free," however please read the labels and see what might be lurking inside of the product.

Also, you should severely limit your use of cheese and dairy. One study I read recently said that everyone had some level of milk allergy. Consider the change to a milk substitute, but I do not recommend "Soy" products as they often are made with GMO grains and will often affect hormone levels.

 I know how hard this is to make these changes, but then stop and think about your motivation. Don't you want to live longer and healthier lives? That is what this book is all about. It is about having <u>health and hope through the use of herbs</u>, but also through taking responsibility for your own body.

What are some herbs other herbs that will strengthen your immune system? Let me suggest a few.

Mushrooms:

Turkey tail (and cancer)

Turkey tail (*Trametes versicolor*) is bracket fungi whose colors and patterns resemble the tail feathers of a turkey.

Turkey tail mushrooms are best known for its cancer fighting properties. One study published in *ISRN Oncology* in 2012, for instance, found that taking up to 9 grams of turkey tail extract per day could improve the immune status of patients with breast cancer. Another study, published one year later in the *International Journal of Molecular Medicine*, discovered that turkey tail, when combined with reishi, another popular disease-fighting mushroom, could induce death in leukemia cells. (NaturalNews.com)

The Reishi mushroom (sometimes Red Reishi)

Christine M. Dionese L.Ac, MSTOM is an integrative health expert writes, "Reishi has multi-faceted immunomodulatory effects. Studies highlight how Reishi can identify potential pathogenic invaders by amplifying natural killer cell activity. Because Reishi's therapeutic action can break down fibrinogen, an outer layer that protects cancer cells, they are more susceptible to cell death." Read more at: http://www.naturalhealth365.com/reishi-mushroom-immune-system-1198.html#sthash.8mhh5pss.dpuf

Lion's mane: cognitive dysfunction

Lion's mane (*Hericium erinaceus*) is a globular-shaped fungus that is easily identified by its cascading teeth-like spines, from which white spores emerge. In fact, the mushroom is also called the "pom-pom blanc" since it resembles the white poms-poms used by cheerleaders.

Lion's mane's positive effects on brain function are well-recorded. For example, a study published in *Biomedical Research* in August 2010 found that subjects who took a lion's mane

supplement for four weeks demonstrated reduced depression and anxiety compared to the placebo group. A review published in *Critical Reviews in Biotechnology* in March 2014 also listed lion's mane as one of
the mushrooms that can prevent age-related neurodegenerative diseases such as Alzheimer's disease and Parkinson's disease.

Sources: (1) Michael Ravensthorpe (www.Spiritfoods.net); http://www.ncbi.nlm.nih.gov

Cordyceps (*Ophiocordyceps sinensis*)

Cordyceps has been shown to be especially useful against lung cancers (in TCM it is said to enter through the Lung meridian). It is also used to increase libido, optimize cholesterol levels, and address liver disease and to relax bronchial tissues, which is helpful for those with certain types of asthma.

If you have breathing issues or bronchial issues this **may** be the herb which will help you. I have had both in the past and I have found that for me, it is better than or just as good as an inhaler with no side effects. I've read that some Olympic athletes use cordyceps to increase their stamina. This is one herb that I personally take daily. **NOTE**: If you are having an episode of breathing problems this is not an instant fix like an inhaler. For me it takes about 20 minutes or more to get into my system and begin to help. After adding this to my diet I have not had those types of breathing issues.

Button Mushroom

"Eating small portions of mushrooms every day can make a big impact on your health. A recent study has found that mushrooms, particularly button mushrooms, contain important antioxidants that fight off chronic diseases, such as dementia, heart disease, and cancer.

To reach this conclusion, researchers from _Pennsylvania State University_ analyzed the relationship between mushroom consumption and the prevalence of chronic disease in people". (NaturalNews.com)

NOTE: Again, let me caution you that I am not a medical doctor, so please consult your doctor before you decide to make these types of changes in your life or health care treatment.

Chapter 9

More boosts for the immune system:

1. Echinacea augustifolia (Latin Genus, species)or Echinacea 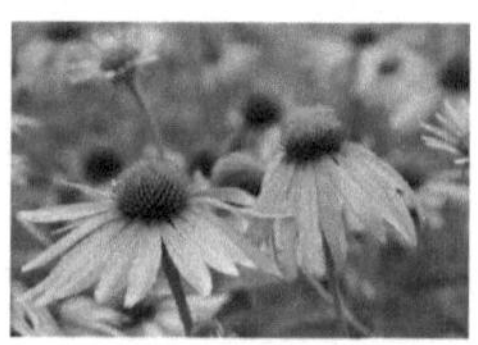 purpurea, more commonly known as Echinacea, is a wondrous plant whose root can aid in providing a healthy immune system. Echinacea strengthens the entire immune system, but don't take it for more than a week at a time, as it loses its effectiveness if you take it for more than 7 days straight. When you start to feel a cold or flu coming on take Echinacea with Vitamin C to knock it out quickly and sometime prevent it from developing at all. But again, note that keeping your immune system healthy is a full time job. You can't just throw some herbs in your body and expect a miracle, (although

it can give you an immediate boost).
It has to be a life style change,
perhaps a change of mindset in
dealing with you health.

Below is part of an article written several
years back **Aurora Geib**

"Foods that boost the body's immune
system can offer a lot of healthy options
for those who wish to be more conscious
in what they take in. To be sustained, the
immune system heavily depends on the
stomach for support. Malnourished
individuals are more susceptible to
disease as opposed to those who observe
a healthy nutritious diet. Below are some
of these examples:

Ginseng - This herb has many varieties.
The most commonly studied variety is
Panax ginseng, also known as Korean
ginseng. Its main active component,
ginsenosides, has been proven to have
anti-inflammatory and anti-cancer
properties. Clinical research studies have
demonstrated that it may improve
immune and psychological functions as
well as conditions related to diabetes.

Garlic - This spice has had a long history of medicinal value. In a recent study conducted by Dr. Ellen Tattelman, an assistant professor at the *Albert Einstein College of Medicine of Yeshiva University*, New York, it was reconfirmed that garlic indeed has cardiovascular, anti-microbial and antineoplastic properties. It's also a perfect spice to use when doing sautéed dishes.

Bell peppers- This pepper variety does not contain capsaicin, unlike its other feisty cousins. On the contrary, it is sweet and crunchy and contains the carotenoid lycopene which lowers the risk of cancer; beta-carotene which is converted to vitamin A; and Zeaxanthin, known to prevent macular degeneration and cataracts.

Ginger - This herb has been shown to reduce inflammation, cardiovascular conditions, blood clots and cholesterol. In a study, researchers found that animal subjects given ginger extracts had a significant reduction in cholesterol and blood clotting qualities. Moreover, it has been observed to inhibit the behavior of genes connected with inflammation.

Turmeric- This spice contains curcumin, which has notable antioxidant properties. It also has antibacterial, anti-inflammatory and stomach soothing benefits. It reduces inflammation by stimulating the adrenal glands to increase the hormone that lessens inflammation. Animal studies on this herb have revealed that turmeric protects the liver from the adverse effects of alcohol and certain toxins. Turmeric also helps in digestive problems by stimulating bile flow.

Gingko Biloba- Gingko biloba's leaves contain antioxidant compounds called bilobalides and ginkgolides that protect the body from damage caused by free radicals. Moreover, it has also been found to protect against radiation. In a study using animal subjects, ginkgo was demonstrated to have protected the test subjects against radiation poisoning. The latest research also suggests that extracts of this herb can neutralize oxidizing agents and free radicals caused in the cells due to radiation, thus preventing cell death. In fact, NaturalNews recently reported that ginkgo extracts reduce brain damage by up to 50 percent.

Astralagus - Also from China, this herb stimulates the immune system and aids in digestion and adrenal gland functions. It is also a diuretic. The effectiveness of this herb is due to polysaccharides, saponins and flavonoids. It has also been taken to combat the common cold and flu. Its digestive health benefits demonstrate the lowering of stomach acidity, resulting to an increase in the body's metabolic rates and the promotion of waste elimination.

Cat's claw - This herb from Peru is commonly used for stomach problems. Recently, however, it is becoming known as an exceptional immune response stimulator that helps the body to fight off infections and degenerative diseases. It contains oxindole alkaloids enhancing the immune system's capacity to engulf and destroy pathogens.

From a practical perspective, taking in food which boosts the immune system while enjoying it at the same time can be a cost effective way to maintain health. Coupled with a healthy lifestyle, sufficient rest and a positive outlook in life, staying healthy does not have to cost an arm and a leg."

NOTE: The entire article can be found at: http://www.immunesystemremedies.com.

I would also add **<u>Andographis</u>**: The bitter make up of andrographis is believed to stimulate the immune system and anti-inflammatory response. Andrographis has been shown to support the immune system against microbial infection.

Chapter 10

A FEW SPECIFIC APPLICATIONS

While it is impossible to address every illness in one book, (and that was not my intent when I began this book), I have received many questions regarding certain health issues and want to touch on a few of them here.

ALLERGIES

Understanding allergies is really complicated, there are thousands of triggers for allergies as you probably know. Sometimes it is impossible to find out exactly what is a person's allergy trigger.

My wife has fought with allergies for years. We grew up and lived in the Central Eastern United States and were told by a Sinus Specialist years ago, the only way to escape the problem is to move to a dry warm climate. Years latter we moved to a dessert area out West and the condition did not improve.

While living in California my wife saw two different allergy specialists. The first did 50 skin test spots which came out inconclusive. He prescribed several allergy medicines, but nothing really seemed to help. About a year latter she saw another specialist that did 100 skin test spots, took 14 vials of blood and had her take an MRI of her sinus. All tests were inconclusive. Again, he prescribed several nasal sprays and allergy medicines.

Bottom line is that nothing they did helped her. I finally convinced her to try a couple of things which I believed would help her. She did and the results were great… *as long as she kept it up she had relief from all of her allergies...* The problem with any treatment (and I know this from my medical doctor friends), is that once someone starts feeling well, they often stop the treatment. It's no different with those who are giving herbal medicine a try.

Here is what we did for her that worked.

First: We stopped almost all dairy products. She did eat some hard cheese and used some "Real" butter, no butter substitutes.

Second: We started her on <u>**Dr. Christopher's Immucalm formula**</u>. One of the problems with which those with allergies are dealing is that their immune system is out of balance, or irritated. Dr. Christopher's formula is designed to do what the name indicates, to Calm the Immune System. You can purchase it through Dr. Christopher's Herb Shop (http://drchristophersherbshop.com/), (phone: 801-489-4500).

> Signs of an overactive immune system include: allergic reactions to certain foods, plants, or animals, or auto-immune diseases. This simple combination of marshmallow root and astragalus has made life easier for those who suffer from allergies, hay fever, and asthma multiple sclerosis, juvenile onset diabetes, rheumatoid arthritis, or any hyperactive immune response. This formula also stimulates the body's ability to fight off infection. (Dr. David Christopher)

If you are having a lot of allergy problems I would recommend you take 2 capsules 2-3 times per day until you get things under control Once your system has calmed down you can take it once a day and see how that works.

Along with this I would advise you to either stop using dairy products completely or at the very least cut back to the bare minimum in use.

Arthritis – What can be done

Arthritis can have several different causes, but the main complaint is the swelling of joints with mineral deposits and the accompanying pain, often making it difficult for them to be used.

One of the problems which we face is the taking in of inorganic material such as calcium and other minerals through Vitamins and mineral supplements. In most areas the water that flows through our taps are filled with inorganic calcium. Just notice all of those deposits around your water taps and in the sinks. These same "Inorganic" materials are often deposited in our joints with no way to rid ourselves of them. Very little inorganic calcium is absorbed into your system, it is deposited by the body as a by product. The thing is, that arthritis can be cured and frozen joints can be made to work again. It may take time, but it can happen if you stay with the program.

Recommendations:

1. My first recommendation is to begin drinking Distilled water which will eliminate one of the main sources of the inorganic minerals. The recommended amounts are 3 quarts for women and 1 gallon per day for men. I personally have never been able to drink that much water, but shoot for at least ½ gallon per day of water and herbal teas. WHY: Because it helps clean out the minerals and other deposits in your system.

2. Also, diet is important. I would recommend that you clean up your diet as much as possible and stop eating foods with damaging additives in them. Stop buying processed (prepared) foods and learn to cook from scratch. Just take a look at the labels on the food you purchase, many of the items listed you can't even pronounce. Are you sure you want to put them into your body. Eliminate milk and dairy products, use Almond milk, I would recommend staying away from Soy milk.

3. Next, using an Apple Cider Vinegar* **"formation"** will be of GREAT benefit. What is a **formation**: Soak a piece of cotton cloth (avoid synthetics) in hot apple cider vinegar and wrap it around the joints. This will ease the pain and aid in dissolving the deposits.

4. Mix - 1 Tablespoon of Apple Cider Vinegar and 1 Tablespoon of organic honey in 8 oz of warm water and drink it at least once a day. It will help dissolve the deposits in the joints.

* **Note**: Purchase Organic Raw – Unfiltered Apple Cider Vinegar. I can recommend the Bragg Brand which is sold in 16 oz bottles in most grocery stores. You will see what is called **"the Mother,"** in the bottle. It is a cloudy mass floating in the vinegar and it is suppose to be there. It is unfiltered and that is one of the things that makes it work well. It has all of the nutrients in it.

Additional Herbal Aids:

***Dr. Christopher's Joint Formula**. This is a combination of herbs that act as a solvent for the calcium deposits. It also contains herbs that relieve pain; herbs rich in organic (easily absorbed) calcium; herbs that kill fungus and infections which sometimes are the cause of the problem.

*Dr. Christopher's **Complete Bone and Tissue** Ointment: This will aid in healing almost any ailment connected to the bones, tissue and muscles.

***NOTE**: These can be Ordered from: Dr. Christopher's Herb Shop on line:

http://www.drchristophersherbshop.com Or Call: 1-800-453-1406

Alzheimer's and Parkinson disease

In an article by Tony Isaac on "Health Secrets," written in 2015, he writes, "Coconut oil for Alzheimer's may be the magic bullet."

He continues, "Naturopaths and other natural health authorities have been telling us for years that coconut oil can not only slow Alzheimer's, it can also stop it and even reverse it. Now, recent science and real life experiences have confirmed what they have told us. With organic coconut oil, you can forget Alzheimer's, it's no longer a death sentence!

Alzheimer's and dementia have been growing at alarming rates thanks to our aging population, widespread use of statin drugs, low fat diets, and the continued inundation of toxins in our food, air and water. It is estimated that the current figure of 5 million plus people with Alzheimer's in the U.S. will triple by 2050. Despite optimistic announcements of advances, mainstream medicine continues to be thwarted at actually finding a cure or reversing Alzheimer's and dementia. The good news, however, is that nature has had an answer all along: coconut oil.

What science has found

According to the researchers, "The rationale for using coconut oil as a potential Alzheimer's Disease therapy is related to the possibility that it could be metabolized to ketone bodies that would provide an alternative energy source for neurons, and thus compensate for mitochondrial dysfunction." (Sayer Ji, Green Medicine Info).

The researchers found that coconut oil protected against amyloid plaque buildup and concluded that "Considering that the medium chain triglyceride found in coconut known as caprylic acid does cross the blood-brain barrier, and has recently been found to have anti-convulsant, in addition to ketogenic effects, coconut oil likely does have a neuroprotective effect."

An in vivo (in the actual body) human study found that brain function was improved after only one dose and study participants reported significant improvements in Alzheimer's disease after 45 and 90 days of treatment with medium chain triglycerides from coconut oil." Sayer Ji, Green Medicine Info).

In another study, Canadian researcher Stephen Cunnane used PET scans to determine that ketones are indeed a possible alternative brain fuel.

Real Life Experiences:

In one of the first widely reported successes with coconut oil, Dr. Mary Newport, MD, dramatically reversed her husband's symptoms of Alzheimer's disease after just two weeks of adding coconut oil to his diet. (https://www.youtube.com/watch?v=Dfux-5Z4COo)

In 2007, a man in England suddenly quickly deteriorated over a one year period to the point that he could barely do anything for himself and he no longer recognized his own daughter. After his son watched the YouTube video of Dr. Mary Newport's success with her husband, they decided to try their father on six tablespoons a day.

"Within a month his mood completely changed," his daughter reported. "He became calmer and relaxed. He started shaving, then bathing on his own. Then one day he gave me a hug and said my name."

<u>Personal Experience:</u>

We have a very good and long time friends who began to fight this battle against dementia. The wife was forgetting things and unable to engage in normal conversation or participate in activities which she formally loved. Her doctor diagnosed her as having early stage dementia. They asked me what I might recommend and I of course told them about the possibilities of using Coconut Oil. I recommended that they buy Coconut oil in capsule form, which my wife and I use daily. She however couldn't swallow the large capsule, so they began using it in its natural state.

Coconut oil can be liquid or a cream similar to butter. Virgin Coconut oil melts at 76 degrees, but remains in a creamy state up until that point. Some people spread it on their toast or of course use it for cooking (much preferred), instead of shorting or other oils. My mother even put it in her hot coco at times. You may say, "I wouldn't like the taste," however coconut oil has almost no taste whatsoever. It does have a coconut fragrance however, so if that bother's you in your cooking, try the capsules.

Prostate: Enlarged (swelling)

The prostate swells due to testosterone. As we age, the testosterone breaks down into Dihydrotestosterone which remains in the prostate and causes the swelling.

Recommendation: Dr. Christopher's *Male Urinary Track Formula*: (available online at Dr. Christopher's Herb Shop). It addresses the results of a swollen prostate **and** is very effective at reducing and dissolving stones in the bladder and kidneys.

Herbs that reduce Prostate swelling:

Saw Palmetto, much better than prescription drugs. It prevents the breakdown of testosterone into Dihydrotestosterone. I have recommended this to friends who have an enlarged prostate and were on prescription meds. They began taking Saw Palmetto and had great results. They actually were able to stop their prescription medicines. (again work with your doctor when trying this). I recommend and use myself a liquid softgel capsule sold by Vitacost,
(https://www.vitacost.com/productResults.as

px?N=0&Ntt=nsi%203006649) which contains Pumpkin Seed Oil also, which makes everything work well together. Pumpkin seeds specific to help with male urinary track. Cleanses and Builds

Personal Experience:

Several years ago my family doctor said my Prostate was slightly enlarged, so I immediately took action, did some research and started on the appropriate herb. I have never had a problem since. I also have a very close personal friend who had a sever problem with an enlarged prostate to the point it was restricting his urine flow. He was on a couple of prescription medications for the problem, but it did not seem to be helping. I recommended the Saw Palmetto with Pumpkin seed oil to him. He told me that in just a few days he started to receive relief. He was able to stop all of his prescription medicine now uses the Saw Palmetto on a daily basis and has no problems.

Chapter 11

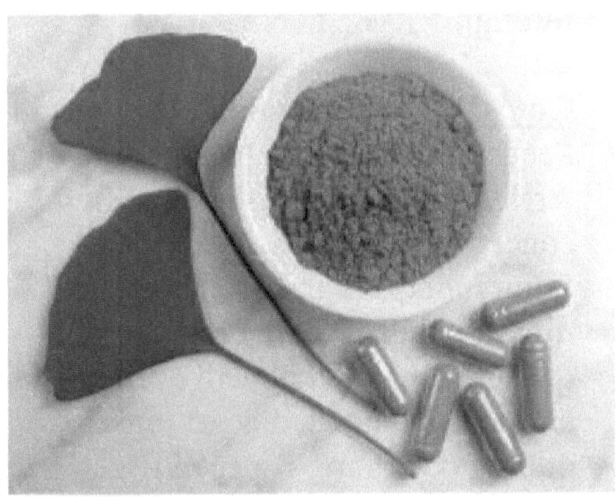

MORE ON HERBS AND MINERALS

Here is a list of what we take daily in order of what I feel is importance to us. (**NOTE**: Do not take pressed powder pills, they do not work well. The body does not dissolve many of these and they pass through your system undisolved, try and stay with powder or liquid filled gelcaps)

1. <u>**Selenium**</u> – General health – Keeps Arteries walls flexible, (I have found this helpful controlling hemorrhoids also), protects from strokes. Fights cancer, helps prevent Cataracts,

fights heart disease, important to the immune system – 200mg (available through Vitacost.com)

2. **<u>CoQ-10</u>** – Heart health, everyone needs this: Relieves Angina, Arrhythmia, Atherosclerosis, fights cancer, relieves congestive heart failure, helps high blood pressure, migraine headaches, Parkinson's disease. This will actually rebuild and repair damaged heart muscle. - 400mg (2-200mg capsules)

3. **<u>L-Arginine</u>** – Reduces cholesterol and cleans arteries, aids in weight loss, decreases angina and congestive heart failure, reduces high blood pressure and arterial disease – 3,600mg (2 – 1,800 mg capsules)

4. **<u>Maca</u>**, a general health booster, gives more energy, increases libido, improves bone density in women – 525mg (one capsule)

5. **<u>Red Rice Yeast</u>** - Reduces cholesterol, fights heart disease, and reduces cancer risk: 1,200 mg (2 capsules) **<u>morning and evening if</u>**

you are having problems with cholesterol.

6. **Flax Seed Oil** – Helps relieve arthritis, fights cancer, and lowers cholesterol, important for brain health. **NOTE:** *Flax Seed Oil acts as a natural blood thinner, do not take if you are on a baby aspirin regimen*. - 2,000mg per day.

7. **Fish Oil** – helps relieve arthritis, asthma and helps protect from cancer, fights cardiovascular disease and much more. **NOTE: We take Vitacost complete EFA, which is a combination of several omega 3 & 6 oils, which are necessary to gain the benefit of the Flax seed Oil.) We take 2 capsules (Vitacost Item number - NSI 3000876)**

8. **Vitamin B Complex** – Important to memory - 100 mg. These essential nutrients help convert our food into fuel, allowing us to stay energized throughout the day.

9. **Glucosamine with Chondroitin & MSM (With Vitamin. C & Manganese)** - Rebuilds cartilage,

fights osteoarthritis, and builds immune system – 1,500 mg.

NOTE: I order this from **Vitacost also. Item #7019274. <u>Dosage</u>:** This kind of depends upon your need, but I take 3 to 6 per day depending upon how my body feels. The more you hurt, the more you increase the dosage. You can take 10-12 per day (throughout the day) if you are having serious problems. Be especially aware that this is not an overnight "healing," but normally you will feel a difference in a few days.

10. **<u>Saw Palmetto</u>** – Helps control prostrate and reduce inflammation or enlargement. (This works VERY well in this area. I have testimonies from several friends who have tried this). Helps prevent hair loss, fights prostrate cancer, for prostrate health, reduces the risk of bladder infection in men and helps control Polycysitc ovarian syndrome in women. -600 mg. (2 capsules daily). Again I order this from Vitacost, but there are other suppliers of good products also.

11. **<u>Cordyceps</u>** – Cordyceps has been shown to be especially useful against lung cancers (in TCM it is said to enter through the Lung meridian). It is also used to increase libido, optimize cholesterol levels, address' liver disease and to relax bronchial tissues, which is helpful for those with certain types of asthma.

If you have breathing issues or bronchial issues this **<u>may</u>** be the herb may help you. I have had both in the past and I have found that for me it is better, or just as good as, an inhaler for me with no side effects. I've read that some Olympic athletes use cordyceps to increase their stamina. This is one herb that I personally take daily.

<u>NOTE:</u> DO NOT STOP USING YOUR INHAILER WITHOUT DISCUSSING THIS WITH YOU MEDICAL PROFESSIONAL.

For me it takes about 20 min for it to kick in, so you don't have the immediate relief of an inhaler, but I take it everyday to strengthen my

lungs and build the immune system. 1,000 mg (2 capsules) (Vitacost Item # - NSI 3001255)

12. **<u>Garlic </u>- Six solid health reasons to use garlic daily** I take at least 3,000 mg per day, (though it is recommended that you take at least 1,000 mg per day.) Reduces cholesterol and cleans arteries, aids in weight loss, decreases angina and congestive heart failure, reduces high blood pressure and is one of the strongest natural antibiotics. This can work as a blood thinner also, so be careful of how much you are taking.

The <u>key medicinal compound in garlic is allicin</u>, which has antibacterial, antiviral, antifungal and antioxidant properties, not to mention all the vitamins and minerals you're getting with garlic, including B1, B6, C, as well as manganese, calcium, copper and selenium. Know that cooking garlic reduces a significant amount of these medicinal qualities. (I recommend using a Liquid filled gelcap. I like Walgreen brand of no odor liquid garlic gelcaps, but have bought them at Wal-Mart recently).

13. **<u>Magnesium</u>** – Helps balance blood sugar, relieves stress and improves sleep, maintains strong bones.

14. **<u>Coconut Oil</u>** – As referenced in this book to keep mentally alert.

Chapter 12

Natural Antibiotics

Goldenseal (*Hydrastis canadensis*): This plant, native to North America, is a traditional treatment for skin infections resulting from scrapes and cuts. The leaf extract is so powerful that it can treat not only minor abrasions, but even superbugs like MRSA – methicillin resistant *Stapholococcus aureus*.

Garlic (*Allium sativum*): While many of us are very familiar with garlic's delicious cooking properties, its powerful medicinal powers are less well known. Garlic is a potent antibacterial when crushed and exposed to air, and laboratory studies have found it as effective as penicillin at treating many infections, though studies on its efficacy against superbug infections is limited

Ginger (*Zingiber officinale*): Ginger is a powerful anti-fungal, anti-viral and antibacterial, and is traditionally used to treat coughs and colds. It has also shown promise in the fight against more serious infections like pneumonia and even superbugs.

Indigo (*Baptisia sp.*): The Indigo plant has proven to be an effective treatment against typhoid. While we do not see many cases of this disease in the U.S., it is interesting to note that typhoid and food-borne salmonella – which does affect about 1 million people each year – are very similar bacteria. It is therefore logical to assume that indigo would also be an effective treatment for cases of salmonella poisoning.

Licorice (*Glycyrrhiza glabra*): This powerful anti-inflammatory is an excellent treatment for allergies and asthma. A word of warning, though: Pregnant women should not consume licorice, and it should be avoided by those with high blood pressure.

Cinnamon (*Cinnamomum zeylanicum*): This well-known spice is an effective treatment for gingivitis as well as other irritations and infections of the mouth.

Honey: Honey is a powerful antibacterial that also speeds up recovery from burns. It can also prevent infection and promote healing. (This is natural, un-pasteurized honey)

Turmeric (*Curcuma longa*): The anti-inflammatory and antimicrobial properties of turmeric make it an effective healer even of wounds that are slow to heal like diabetic wounds and pressure ulcers. It is most effective when used as an ointment.

Elderberry (*Sambucus nigra*): Elderberry boosts immunity, making the body better able to fight off any infection and helping to avoid the necessity for antibiotics.

Echinacea (*Echinacea purpura*): Studies have found that Echinacea (Purple Cone Flower roots), is at least as effective as pharmaceutical anti-viral drugs in the treatment of the common flu. Patients who take Echinacea have been found to suffer fewer complications and side effects than those treated with anti-virals.

Cumin (*Cuminum cyminum*): This well-known Middle Eastern spice is a powerful antimicrobial, and can treat mouth infections that even antibiotics are useless against. It is likely, therefore, that it would be effective against superbugs.

Cranberries: Cranberries contain anti-inflammatory properties which mean they can both prevent and treat urinary tract infections (UTIs). By preventing bacteria from sticking to the walls of the bladder, cranberries also help to prevent recurring bladder infections. (These descriptions by Rebecca Tarrant, writing for *Ask a Prepper*).

Note: If you are drinking Cranberry Juice from the local grocery store you are probably wasting your money. Most of it has so much sugar or high fructose corn syrup in it that it negates any benefit you might have received. Again, check out the labels and perhaps pay a visit to your local health food store for the right kind of juice.

Coconut Oil: "The benefits of coconut oil is due to the presence of lauric, capric, and caprylic acids in it and the antimicrobial, antioxidant, antifungal, and antibacterial properties inherent within the oil. Our bodies convert the lauric acid into monolaurin, which fights the viruses and bacteria associated with herpes, flu, HIV, listeria, and giardia". (Hesh Goldstein)

A REQUST FOR YOU:

Each of us who are Amazon Kindle Authors struggle to make our way in the thousands of book provided here. **It would really; really** help if you could take a few minutes and leave feedback in the "**Write a Customer Review**" section on my book page. (It's to the right of the box with the stars on the top).

Thanks in advance for your help!
Russ Lawson

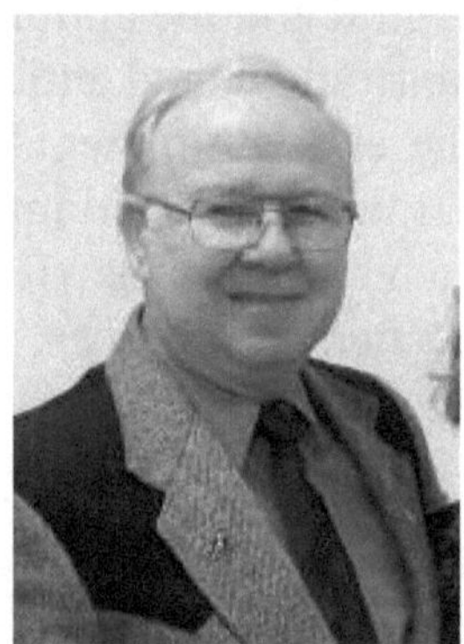

Russ Lawson

Some Resources for you

<u>WEBSITES:</u>

<u>Health, Hope and Herbs</u> website, (My site which is always growing and has new blog entries on a continual basis. Has good information and links to other sites)

<u>School of Natural Healing</u> (Herbal school website, everything you want to know about further learning in Herbal Medicine.)

<u>American Youngevity</u> (Liquid Minerals and many other supplements)

<u>www.supralife.com</u> (Supplements)

<u>http://www.drchristophersherbshop.com</u> or by calling (888) 327-4372. (A great source of prepared and proven natural compounds, herbs and books)

<u>http://www.chrisbeatcancer.com</u> (Website of someone else that has fought the battle and won. Lots of links and information)

<u>http://naturalnews.com</u> (One of my favorite informational websites. They feature lots of

writers from all over the world and products to help you live healthy lives)

http://Vitacost.com (Where I buy many of my herbs and supplements. Has good prices and good products. I especially like the customer review section, much like Amazon.)

BOOKS

Herbal Medicine: Is it the right choice for you?
This book was written to build people's confidence in the fact that Herbs can really help make their lives better. I want them to understand that all herbs are not "Snake Oil", or "Grandma's old potions," but real medicine that really helps.

Dr. Mom's Health Living (Though pricy at $27.00, this is one of my favorite Herbal Medicine books and more detailed than many. She deals with many illnesses and herbal cures and gives details about treatment).

Herbal Home Health Care, Dr. David Christopher, (This excellent reference volume lists diseases in convenient alphabetical order with concise definitions, symptom descriptions, causes, and herbal aids, other natural treatments, the incurables program, detoxification and the mucusless diet. A book for every family)

Eat to live, by Dr. Joel (Hailed a "medical breakthrough" by Dr. Mehmet Oz, EAT TO LIVE offers a highly effective, scientifically proven way to lose weight quickly. The key to Dr. Joel Fuhrman's revolutionary six-week plan is simple: health = nutrients / calories. When the ratio of nutrients to calories in the food you eat is high, you lose weight. The more nutrient-dense food you eat, the less you crave fat, sweets, and high-caloric foods.)

Resources Cited in this book

<u>Health, Hope and Herbs</u> website,
My <u>unexpected adventure</u> website
WebMD.com
www.radiologyinfo.org
http://waytogonutrition.com/eyology.htm
<u>School of Natural Healing</u> (Herbal school website)
<u>American Youngevity</u> (Liquid Minerals)
www.supralife.com
http://www.drchristophersherbshop.com or by calling (888) 327-4372.
http://www.chrisbeatcancer.com
<u>Science Translational Medicine.</u>
http://www.nature.com
http://www.bbc.co.uk
http://lpi.oregonstate.edu
http://science.naturalnews.com
<u>The Healing Factor</u>;
<u>Cancer and Vitamin C</u>
http://www.naturalhealth365.com
http://cancerisover.blogspot.com
http://www.alive.com
http://treatmentcancercells.com
http://www.carrotmuseum.co.uk
http://healthmaven.blogspot.com
http://www.naturalhealth365.com/reishi-mushroom-immune-system-1198.html#sthash.8mhh5pss.dpuf

www.Spiritfoods.net
http://www.ncbi.nlm.nih.gov
Fight off chronic diseases
Pennsylvania State University
http://www.immunesystemremedies.com(htt
ps://www.youtube.com/watch?v=Dfux-
5Z4COo – Video on coconut oil and
Alzheimer's
Anti-inflammatory and antimicrobial
properties of turmeric
Ask a Prepper website
WebND
Sayer Ji, Green Medicine Info, Author
Hesh Goldsteind, Author

Other Books by this author on Kindle:

<u>Natural Cure for Cancer</u>
The doctors said it was cancer, but I refused to accept standard treatment and discovered Herbal Medicine offered me answers and a cure.

<u>Herbal Medicine: Is it the right choice for you?</u>
This book was written to build people's confidence in the fact that Herbs can really help make their lives better. I want them to understand that all herbs are not "Snake Oil", or "Grandma's old potions," but real medicine that really helps.

<u>A dog size hole in your heart!</u>
Russ has tried to put on paper his and his wife's experiences with their three fur babies. Each of their deaths was a deep and painful experience emotionally. They grieved, but learned to deal with the losses.

This book was written to try and help others understand that they are not alone in their special grief. They are not strange or weird, they are caring people who love deeply and that is as it should be. It walks you through the steps we must go through to deal with grieving over the loss of our pets.

<u>Back Pain Relief</u>
The authors back injury led him on a journey of discovery to find relief.

<u>Words of hope for desperate times</u>
Are you feeling down or discouraged, this book will lift your spirits and give you a new look at your life and God.

<u>Is God Mad at me? (Why is bad stuff happening).</u>

<u>Missions the real deal!</u>
What is life like living on a mission field in Africa? This book journals our lives in this challenging work.

<u>Elders and Deacons in the church</u>
A study of God's leadership in His church.

<u>More stories to touch the heart</u>
Stories of encouragement from life that will lift your spirit.

Special Request:

I'm asking that you take a few minutes and leave a review of this book. As an independent author my listing on Amazon is determined by the reviews I receive. If you found what I had to say interesting or informative, please give me a positive review.

Thank You,
Russ Lawson